Paleo for Beginners

Lose Weight and Get Healthy with the Paleo Diet, Including a 21 Paleo Diet Recipes and 7-Day Meal Plan Solution

Sarah Sparrow

I0439422

PUBLISHED BY:
Sarah Sparrow
Copyright © 2013

Table of Contents

Chapter 1: Introduction to the Paleo Diet

Welcome to a new way of eating and living that has helped many individuals lose weight, increase their energy and feel good all-around for the first time in many years. While the Paleo Diet is not new, the hype and attention it has been receiving over the past few years has brought it to the forefront of nutritional websites, morning news shows and fitness blogs. Whether you are reading this to learn more about the diet, decide if it's the right way of living for you, or have already committed and just need a little guidance, you've come to the right place! Getting started with the Paleo Diet is designed with you in mind. It is an attempt to dissect the diet into relatable chunks so that you can be a fully informed caveman or woman!

Every individual that considers the Paleo Diet does so for different reasons. Whether you are facing serious health problems and trying a homeopathic approach, needing to lose weight, or would simply like to run around with your children and not get winded, then the Paleo Diet is a good starting place.

Below, you'll find some answers to the questions that you might be thinking about when considering the Paleo Diet. You'll be given an overview of the Paleo Diet before it is further dissected in the coming chapters, a brief history of the diet and a summary of the science behind the idea that has revolutionized and improved the lives of thousands of men and women. Welcome to Getting Started With The Paleo Diet!

What is the Paleo Diet?

The Paleo Diet isn't so much a diet as it is a complete overhaul of the way that you eat. The word diet often brings to mind restriction and calorie counting. So many people have found the Paleo Diet to be helpful because there is none of that within this way of eating. Millions have picked up the Paleo Diet because you are basically learning how to eat and appreciate real food. The only sacrifice you make is purging your home of unwanted calories and replacing them with real, grown-from-the-ground fruits and vegetables, lean meats ideally purchased from a local farm and fresh seafood. Let me explain.

Much like the name suggests, followers of the Paleo Diet believe that the human race functions best when we eat like our Paleolithic cavemen forefathers. They model their eating after the hunter-gatherer society of old, relying on plenty of fruits, vegetables, nuts, berries, seafood and lean meats to supply all of the nutrients their body needs. Being suspicious of the Industrial Revolution, they forgo any and all processed carbohydrates like cereal, pasta, whole grains and candy. They focus their eating on clean foods and try to eat organic as much as possible.

The History of the Paleo Diet

The Paleo Diet hasn't always been as popular as it is today. Partly in thanks to the rise in the philosophy of fitness known as Cross Fit, more and more people are following the Paleo Diet but that hasn't always been the case. In the beginning it was just one lone man named Dr. Loren Cordain.

Dr. Cordain's interest in Paleolithic eating came during his college years. He had always been an athlete and began to devour anything related to athletic performance and diet. He went on to receive a PhD in health from the University of Utah in 1981 and continued to form his nutritional beliefs. After reading a paper by Dr. Boyd Eaton in the New England Journal of Medicine in 1985 about "Paleolithic Nutrition" he was hooked on the concept.

Fast forward to 2002 when his life's work The Paleo Diet was first published. Athletes all over the world found his arguments compelling and regular men and women who needed to lose weight found amazing results once they began to follow his principles. As science progressed he released a new edition in 2010 that is the recommended version for readers.

Although Cordain was the founder, a man named Rob Wolf took the Paleo Diet and was determined to get the idea out to the masses. Wolf, a former research biochemist, personally experienced amazing health and weight loss results once he cut out refined foods, trans fat and sugar. He continued to spread the love around his Cross Fit gym and saw the health of his gym members improve. Diabetes went away, blood pressure and cholesterol were lowered and couples overcame infertility issues just by eating clean and healthy. He even found that people suffering from autoimmune diseases experienced significant improvement when on the diet.

Wolf worked to slowly make the Paleo Diet a household name. He published The Paleo Solution: The Original Human Diet in 2010 that included a foreword by Loren Cordain. His book became a New York Times Bestseller and made the Paleo Diet a force with which to be reckoned. He has gone on to offer podcasts on the subject and travels all around the world to teach men and women how to follow the Paleo Diet.

How does the Paleo diet work?

Hopefully your interest has been peaked and you are now wondering about the science behind this popular diet and lifestyle change. We will attempt to explain this in a simple way and offer further resources for those of you who want to keep learning. To begin let's go back to that original paper written by Dr. Eaton in the New England Journal of Medicine in 1985. Eaton claimed that in the last 40,000 years human genetic constitution has experienced very little change. Even though the invention of agriculture and the Industrial Revolution have occurred, there is no strong scientific evidence that this has changed the evolutionary makeup of the human body. Dr. Cordain would later write that in 40,000 years the human genome has changed less than 0.02%. To put it simply, the way we make food has changed; the way our bodies digest and use this food has not.

A logical connection for Paleo scientists is that, quite literally, the food we eat is killing us. Before civilization began, nature provided all of the foods that were both necessary and helpful for our bodies to consume. It is the human race that is responsible for chemically altering and processing food to the point where it actually becomes unhealthy for us to continue to consume most mass-produced food items.

In October 2011 Rainer J. Klement and Ulrike KŠmmerer published a paper in the journal Nutrition & Metabolism titled, Is there a role for carbohydrate restriction in the treatment and prevention of cancer? Their results provided further proof our bodies are simply not wired for so much grain consumption. According to the scientists, grains increase the risk of inflammation because they are high in omega-6 fatty acids, lectins and gluten. Perhaps the greatest support for the Paleo Diet was found in their final analysis. When they looked at individuals on diets low in fat but rich in whole grains, they were unable to control and reduce cardiovascular health issues on the same par as followers of the Paleo Diet.

The Paleo Diet food pyramid is simple to follow. There is no calorie counting or keeping track of consumed fat grams. It allows for proteins found in meat, fish, poultry and eggs. Carbohydrates come naturally from fruits and vegetables low in starch and sugar. You can eat large quantities of healthy fats that are found in nature. This includes, but is not limited to, healthy oils like coconut oil and avocado oil, nuts, seeds, ghee, grass-fed butter and nut butters such as almond or cashew butter. Any snacks that you consume are not usually opened from a box but made from the list of approved ingredients.

The Paleo Diet works because it is stripping your body of all unnecessary processed foods and filling it with nutritionally packed ingredients. While it might seem like a radical adjustment in the beginning, you will begin to notice changes relatively quickly as your body efficiently uses the fuel you are giving it to become as nature intended – happy and healthy.

Chapter 2: The Characteristics of the Paleo Diet

Because the Paleo Diet requires a drastic change in the way that most people eat an initial food shock usually occurs. It tends to go against many mainstream-dieting beliefs and requires the participant to be open-minded and willing to accept that many traditional modes of eating healthy are simply missing the mark. The characteristics of the Paleo Diet involve: higher protein intake, higher healthy fat intake of monounsaturated and polyunsaturated fats, lower carbohydrate intake and a much higher intake of fruits and vegetables. To begin, let's look at the importance of protein.

Protein

If you are a carnivore, then you will love the Paleo Diet as proteins found in healthy meat and seafood make up the backbone of the diet. If we look at the role that protein plays in your body then you will understand why the Paleo Diet places such a high importance on high quality sources of protein.

Protein is the basic building block that provides cell structure. Words like enzymes and amino acids are specialized words for proteins that provide important functions when it comes to nutrition. Proteins are responsible for proper digestion, communication that occurs within your body, muscle movement and cell reproduction. A diet high in protein assures that your body is getting the essential amino acids that it needs to stay healthy and strong.

Because protein is such an important part of our diet, it ideally should come from a source that values the animal. If an animal is raised free-range and allowed to graze and wander as nature intended, the meat that it produces will be full of healthy and beneficial nutrients like vitamin D, omega-3 and omega-6 fats. Once you begin to eat healthy meat found in humanely raised animals you will begin to feel and see the difference.

Fat

One of the biggest hurdles for traditional dieters to overcome when adopting the Paleo Diet is accepting the belief that good fat does NOT make you fat. That is worth repeating: good fat does not make you fat. The problem with most of our diets is that we are consuming horrible fats. So when nutritionists urge us to have low-fat diets they are right! They simply need to insert the word "bad" into their slogan. We need to purge our diets of bad fats and learn what fats will keep our bodies healthy.

Just as important as meat is in the Paleo Diet, so, too, are the fat sources that create a foundation for the diet. One of the most well-known uses of body fat is energy. Fats also make tissue and create important things like hormones. Your lungs are coated with saturated fats and your liver needs saturated fat to function properly. But not all fats are created equally.

The Paleo Diet is high in saturated fat. Saturated fat helps to reduce bad cholesterol (known as LDL) and raise good cholesterol (HDL). This is why foods like butter, tallow, and lard are encouraged. They contain plenty of soluble vitamins like A, D, E and K that can only be absorbed by the body with the help of healthy fats. In addition to saturated fat, the medium-chain fatty acids (MCFAs) found in coconut oil is also recommended.

Coconut oil has been called the tropics best kept secret because it is packed with healthy saturated fat and MCFAs that your liver can use for immediate energy. MCFAs are also referred to as medium-chain triglycerides (MCTs) and activate something pretty cool inside the body when you eat them: they boost your metabolism and signal your body to use fat for energy instead of storing it as fat and stacking on the pounds!

The main point about fats is this: there are good fats and bad fats. Bad fats or unsaturated fats (like vegetable oil and canola oil) make your body feel sluggish and promote fat storage. Good fats, or saturated fats (like coconut oil), keep your body lean and strong and promote fat for energy.

Carbohydrates

Many people who adopt the Paleo Diet and try to explain it to friends and family will often hear, "So it's like the Atkins Diet?" Well, not really. Yes, the Paleo Diet is low in carbohydrates but a specific type. The Paleo Diet discourages refined sugars and grains, high-glycemic carbohydrates and processed foods.

While sugar is scrumptious to consume, your body pays dearly for the enjoyment. It causes your blood glucose levels to go on a roller coaster ride. This is why you can eat a donut and coffee for breakfast and feel fine…for a few hours. Then the headache sets in, you start to feel lethargic and so you grab a granola bar. The cycle starts all over again. Instead of providing your body with healthy long lasting energy found in good fats and proteins, it is constantly being fed small amounts of sugar that it gives it a momentary rush. Sugar is also very low in nutrients and can legitimately cause addiction if you consume too much.

Grains are another no-no on the Paleo Diet and can be a difficult one for many to adopt. Since traditional nutritional touts the benefits of whole grains, many people look at the Paleo Diet and scratch their heads. Why would things like quinoa, barley and rye be discouraged?

Many grains are high in gluten, a type of protein found in most grains. This protein is incredibly difficult for the body to digest. In some ways, gluten works against your intestines and can actually prevent the intestines from keeping unwanted substances away from your bloodstream. Grains are also high in phytic acid, which prevents absorption of essential minerals. Lectins are nutrients found in most grains that can irritate your digestive system. The list can go on and on of why the grain revolution might have made food production easier, but it did nothing to help our bodies!

High glycemic carbohydrates cause a rapid rise in the body's glucose levels. Remember that roller coaster ride we talked about? A diet containing high glycemic carbohydrates will leave your body lethargic and oftentimes feeling bloated. Foods like white bread, bagels and puffed rice contain this type of carbohydrate. Since the goal is to establish controlled blood sugar levels and few insulin spikes, most Paleo eaters stay away from high glycemic carbohydrates.

Processed foods are discouraged for all the reasons listed above! They are filled with high glycemic carbohydrates, refined sugars and grains. They are simply bad for you because they are created with bad ingredients. It's best to stick with healthy foods and throw away the boxes, bags and tubes of processed junk.

Fruits and Vegetables

If we can't get our carbohydrates from traditional sources, then how does someone on the Paleo Diet get enough carbohydrates to stay healthy and strong? The answer comes from nature: fruits and vegetables. While it is true that a Paleo Diet will be lower in carbohydrates than a traditional diet, followers still receive more than enough carbohydrates from the fruits and vegetables that they consume. Foods like sweet potatoes, vegetables and fruits contain just the right amount of non-processed carbohydrates that will provide your body with all of the necessary nutrients and energy it needs.

Hopefully you have gained a greater understanding of why the Paleo diet labels some foods healthy and others taboo. The key to the Paleo diet is to think clean and natural. If you have to read through a list of twenty ingredients to figure out what's in that cheese puff, then chances are it's not that good for you! Eventually you will enjoy the simplicity of the diet and find that eating healthy fats, proteins and carbohydrates will increase your health and deepen your satisfaction.

Chapter 3: Benefits of the Paleo Diet

Now that you have a greater grasp on the nutrition behind the diet, let's talk a little about the benefits that can come with the Paleo Diet. Men and women have experienced some pretty great results and are living healthier lives just by changing a few basic things about the way they eat. The Paleo Diet can help with weight loss, disease prevention, over-all health improvement and increased energy levels.

Weight Loss

It should come as no surprise that when you cut out the bad foods that are making you tired, sick and bloated, and start consuming healthy, natural, clean foods, your body will experience some drastic results. While weight loss isn't the goal of the Paleo Diet, it certainly is an added benefit. If, however, you are approaching the Paleo Diet from a weight loss standpoint, you will need to make a few modifications.

Paleo for weight loss can be tricky because you are not counting calories. That doesn't mean that calories are thrown out the window, but it does mean that you are focusing on the quality of the calories you are consuming as opposed to stressing out over the quantity. Will you lose weight if you eat a 1200 calories diet of Cheetos? Sure! But your body will feel horrible.

For most people facing obesity, their bodies are experiencing an overload of carbohydrates. Instead of eating a balanced diet of healthy proteins, fats and carbohydrates, they are dining on potato chips, granola bars and pizza, and their insulin and leptin levels are going crazy. Instead of eating foods that are high in fat and can be burned as energy, they are pumping crazy levels of glycogen from empty carbohydrates into their system. The body becomes so overloaded that it stores the extra calories as fat.

Because your body is significantly out of whack (to use a less scientific term) beginning the Paleo Diet with weight loss in mind is a little different than someone who is already at a healthy weight level. If trying to lose weight, focus on fat and stay away from starchier carbohydrates like potatoes. Pump your body full of good fat and nutrient dense vegetables but limit even your natural sugar intake found in fruits. The best ways to lose weight on the Paleo Diet is to meet with a licensed nutritionist who believes in the Paleo Diet and create a meal plan that works for your weight loss goals.

Disease Prevention

While there is no guarantee that following the Paleo Diet will give you a clean pass to all diseases, it will increase your overall health and decrease the chances of finding yourself in the doctor's office with some heartbreaking news. Even though healing of diseases will not necessarily occur, there are certain types of diseases that do see significant improvement. Individuals with autoimmune diseases and digestive problems have seen a decrease in symptoms while on the Paleo Diet.

Because autoimmune diseases are related to your digestive system, it is only natural that the Paleo Diet would work to decrease symptoms. If you are following the Paleo Diet to heal your autoimmune disease, there are specific guidelines that you must follow. Chances are your intestines have become permeable, meaning larger particles that are meant to stay in the intestines are allowed to enter the bloodstream and cause all kinds of problems. We call this, in very scientific terms, leaky gut.

If trying to mend the damage caused by gluten, dairy, stress or inflammation, the Paleo Diet will work with some restrictions. It is best to stay away from nuts and seeds, vegetables that fall in the nightshade family and egg whites.

Improved Health

When the Paleo Diet is functioning properly, your body will become an efficient fat burning machine! Removing all of the junk from your diet will allow your body to function as nature intended. Possibly for the first time in your life you will wake up and know what it's like to just feel good.

It would be impossible to list all of the health benefits of the Paleo Diet so we'll deal with some of the most common.

Measurably, the Paleo Diet can lower cholesterol and lower high blood pressure. Your body will feel consistently good, as insulin and blood sugar levels are kept constant. Followers of the diet experience fewer headaches, fewer sick days and wake up ready to go!

Increased Energy Levels

Our bodies were made to hunt, gather, forage and build. Our ancestors were not sedentary people; their days were spent in the busy process of survival. Modern man has some obstacles to overcome. Our lives are more sedentary and we have to seek recreation to achieve what naturally happened for our caveman forefathers. Instead of being surrounded with healthy, growing foods in season, we find ourselves overloaded with an abundance of both healthy and unhealthy options.

If we consider the idea that maybe, just maybe, our bodies have not changed that much since the Paleolithic era, and then we're open to the possibility that stripping down our food to the very basics once again makes sense. When you put nutrient-dense foods into your body it literally eats it up! What the body doesn't need comes out as waste, not stored as unnecessary fat. Like a car after a much-needed tune-up, a body on the Paleo Diet has the necessary energy stores to keep it going.

If you are trying to lose weight, get an autoimmune disease under control or just desire to feel better than you do today, then the Paleo Diet might be able to help. With countless testimonials and real stories of changed lives, followers of the Paleo Diet are proof that it does work. If you are facing any of these concerns, the best thing to do is talk with your doctor or nutritionist to create a Paleo Diet plan that will increase your quality of life and bring energy back into your day.

Chapter 4: Foods to eat and not to eat

Now that we've discussed the benefits of the Paleo Diet, talked about what sets the diet apart from some of the more popular options, and given a basic overview, it's time to get down to specifics. By now you might be asking yourself, "What can I eat?" That's a great question because it has a wonderful answer!

What can I eat?

On the Paleo Diet you will be feasting on lamb, beef, chicken and pork. You will find yourself consuming seafood with delicious cream sauces and vegetables that are seasoned to perfection. When it gets right down to it, Paleo is more about opening your world of food than closing it off.

Let's begin with the good stuff. Here's a categorized lists of food that are encouraged on the Paleo Diet:

Proteins (to name a few)

- Beef   (preferably grass fed)
    - ❖ Steaks
    - ❖ Ground
    - ❖ Jerky
    - ❖ Veal

- Seafood (preferably wild-caught)
    - ❖ Salmon
    - ❖ Tuna
    - ❖ Red Snapper
    - ❖ Bass
    - ❖ Halibut
    - ❖ Mackerel
    - ❖ Tilapia
    - ❖ Swordfish
    - ❖ Trout
    - ❖ Walleye

- Chicken (preferably pastured and organic)
    - ❖ Thighs
    - ❖ Legs
    - ❖ Wings
    - ❖ Breast

- Pork
    - ❖ Tenderloin
    - ❖ Chops
    - ❖ Bacon (nitrate free)

- Lamb
- Eggs
- Wild Game (deer, rabbit, buffalo, etc.)
- Turkey

Carbohydrates (to name a few)

- Fruits (fresh and frozen)

    - ❖ Apples
    - ❖ Avocados
    - ❖ Bananas
    - ❖ Blackberries

- ❖ Blueberries
- ❖ Cantaloupe
- ❖ Figs
- ❖ Grapefruit
- ❖ Grapes
- ❖ Kiwi
- ❖ Lemon
- ❖ Lime
- ❖ Mango
- ❖ Oranges
- ❖ Papaya
- ❖ Peaches
- ❖ Plums
- ❖ Raspberries
- ❖ Strawberries
- ❖ Tangerines
- ❖ Tomatoes
- ❖ Watermelon

- Vegetables (fresh and frozen)
  - ❖ Artichokes
  - ❖ Asparagus
  - ❖ Avocado
  - ❖ Beets
  - ❖ Broccoli
  - ❖ Brussels Sprouts
  - ❖ Cabbage
  - ❖ Cauliflower
  - ❖ Carrots
  - ❖ Celery
  - ❖ Eggplant
  - ❖ Garlic
  - ❖ Greens (Arugula, Spinach, Kale, Chard, Mustard Greens, Bok Choy, etc.)
  - ❖ Green Onions
  - ❖ Peppers (all varieties)
  - ❖ Squash (all varieties)
  - ❖ Zucchini

❖ Yams
- Fresh Herbs

Fats

- Olive Oil
- Olives
- Coconut Oil
- Coconut Milk
- Unsweetened Coconut Flakes
- Coconut Butter
- Nuts (in moderation)
- Clarified Grass-fed Butter
- Avocado Oil

Non-Perishables

- Canned Tomatoes
- Vinegars (balsamic, apple cider, etc.)
- Stocks (Chicken, Beef, Vegetable)
- Mustard
- Coconut Flour
- Sea Salt
- Pepper
- Variety of Herbs and Spices

What about calcium?

While this list has some wonderful, mouth-watering ingredients, you probably noticed that there are several items that are missing. Specifically, the food group often labeled Dairy is nowhere to be found. There are several views on this so keep reading.

Because those who lived during the Paleolithic era did not consume dairy at all, it has been a source of tension among the Paleo Diet community. Those who adhere to strict Paleo have completely eliminated milk from their diets (except, of course, breast milk in infancy).

However, just because our ancestors did not consume something isn't necessarily the basis for kicking it out of your diet. For others who totally abstain or limit their dairy intake, it has more to do with both the positives and negatives of dairy consumption. Positively, the right kind of dairy can bring good bacteria into your stomach. Fermented dairy products like kefir are a great way to get the benefits of probiotics minus the sugar as it disappears during the process of fermentation. This brings us to the negative aspect of dairy: lactose.

The simplest way to define lactose is to call it milk sugar. For some people, after they consume dairy products heavy in lactose, they may get diarrhea, feel bloated or experience gas. None of these responses make you feel good! In addition to lactose, dairy products can also be high in carbohydrates and can affect insulin levels.

The best way to determine if you have lactose sensitivity is to simply cut it out of your diet. There is nothing in dairy or milk (including Vitamin D and calcium) that you cannot get somewhere else. If you remove dairy from your diet for a month and do not notice a change, then you can always start consuming it once again. If, however, you cut out dairy and notice that you are less bloated, less gassy and have regular bowel movements, then you might have found the hidden gem that was making you feel less than 100%.

Part of the fear of completely cutting out dairy from your diet is found in one little word: calcium. It is legitimate to be concerned about your calcium levels. Calcium is essential to healthy teeth and bones. Calcium helps our blood clots, conducts nerve impulses and aids muscle contraction and relaxation. The easiest way for nutritionists and doctors to get calcium into their patients is through milk.

If, however, you are not consuming milk but are eating plenty of healthy vegetables, then your calcium levels should be fine. Arguably they will be even better as the lining of your gut heals and can then absorb more calcium! For example, one cup of cooked Spinach has almost as much calcium as a cup of milk. The same goes for two cups of cooked broccoli. If you are following the Paleo Diet as intended and greedily gobbling up a variety of vegetables, then your calcium levels should be just fine. If you do choose to consume dairy, then here's a quick list of dairy that's considered the best choices for those trying to follow the Paleo Diet:

- 100% Full Fat Cream
- Raw, Grass-Fed Cheese
- Full Fat Greek Yogurt
- Kefir

In addition to dairy, here are some common foods that are NOT allowed on the Paleo Diet:

- Hotdogs
- Deli Meat
- Ham
- Spam
- Peanuts (they are actually legumes, not nuts)
- Soft Drinks
- Fruit Juices
- Legumes
- Grains
- Energy Drinks
- Sweets

As you can imagine from looking at this list, this isn't your typical open a box, add some meat and (voila!) here's dinner. The Paleo Diet opens up the world of cooking to its adherents. The majority of foods on the Paleo Diet require some prep time. They force you to step into your kitchen and chop fruits, sauté vegetables and make sauces from scratch to pour over succulent cuts of meat.

If you are new to cooking, don't let this scare you! The foods you will be consuming are delicious; it will just take some time to readjust your pallet to enjoy foods as they were meant to taste. If you are used to eating a turkey sandwich and potato chips everyday for lunch, you will have to get used to a fresh salad with chicken, beets, sautéed onions and a balsamic and oil dressing.

But, once you do, there is no going back to the ways of old.

What about salt?

The final thing worth mentioning here is the usage of salt in the Paleo Diet. Across the board everyone agrees that a diet low in salt is good for you. Let me rephrase that: very good for you. The reality, however, is that most of us get such huge amounts of salt from processed foods (including processed meats) and our never ending urges to dine out. When cooking at home you will naturally use less salt as you are adding salt for flavor, not preservation. Unless you have health concerns, adding salt in moderation should be fine. Just be sure to choose unprocessed sea salts.

Chapter 5: Getting Started with the Diet

Now that we've explained all the ins and outs of the Paleo Diet, you might still be left with some questions. The decision to take on the Paleo Diet can be complicated especially if you have specific health issues or there are specific situations in your family that need to be addressed. Here's a simple FAQ's section to try and answer some common questions that arise.

How is the Paleo Diet different from other diets?

There are two main differences of the Paleo Diet: you are not counting calories and you are consuming high levels of good fats. The Paleo Diet is also fairly restrictive when it comes to processed foods, as it believes there is more to staying healthy and fit than simply tracking calories going in and calories being burned. On the Paleo Diet, the quality of what you are consuming is more important than the quantity. You are not tracking points, counting calories or weighing chicken breasts; you are learning how to eat and enjoy real food!

Is it another fad diet?

At its heart the Paleo Diet is not a diet at all. It is more like a lifestyle of eating. The Paleo Diet is trying to educate people, one household at a time, on the value of consuming fresh, clean foods that are good for your overall health.

Is the Paleo Diet safe?

As the Paleo Diet has risen in popularity, many nutritionists have come out against the diet. The main complaints about the diet are as follows: total elimination of dairy that can lead to low calcium levels, lack of whole grains, high animal protein which could lead to increased cholesterol levels and, outside of safety issues, seems expensive and impractical over the long-term.

We have answered the issues of dairy and whole grains so let's talk a little bit about the Paleo Diet and cholesterol. Just as you need to adjust your view of fat you also need to adjust your view of cholesterol. Our bodies are loaded with cholesterol and actually need it to survive. We need the good type of cholesterol known as HDL (as opposed to the bad LDL cholesterol).

One of the main ways that cholesterol works to help the body is during periods of inflammation. When our arteries become inflamed due to high levels of insulin (that have come about from too many carbohydrates) then cholesterol comes to the rescue to heal the inflammation. Once it gets the job done, it should leave the arteries. The only problem is that it doesn't. It doesn't leave the arteries because there is so much inflammation that more cholesterol is needed and the vicious cycle begins. It is here we see that cholesterol is not bad; the inflammation from unhealthy foods is the problem.

At the end of the day it's a personal decision as to whether or not the diet will work for your lifestyle. It does go against many modern medicines because it looks at the body holistically and tries to heal it naturally before turning to medical treatments.

Is the Paleo Diet okay for diabetics?

Diabetes is a rising epidemic in countries all over the world. Many have even called it the disease of the modern era because our diets are nutritionally poor and we lead rather sedentary lives.

Unlike our ancestors, we are not constantly on the move, consuming organic meat and vegetables to keep us alive.

When an individual is diagnosed with diabetes, the first thing that should happen (if they really want to manage and/or heal their disease) is to sit in front of a nutritionist. The nutritionist will typically give them a copy of whatever government food guide is in circulation and create a meal plan around those recommendations. The problem with the food guide is that it is still encouraging them to eat way too many carbohydrates and discouraging them from consuming healthy fats resulting to very little changes.

The Paleo Diet is more than okay for diabetics; it's what nature intended! Paleo reduces the unhealthy carbohydrates that encourage insulin resistance and helps to get your insulin levels on track. It repairs your gut lining to reduce inflammation and gut permeability. It also emphasizes eating healthy foods and naturally restricting your sugars.

If you are diabetic and trying to eat Paleo, then you should make a few modifications to your diet that a traditional Paleo Dieter wouldn't have to make. The main issue is the amounts of fruits that you consume, as these are your primary source of sugar while on the diet. It might be best to limit the amounts of fruits you eat and stay away from dried fruits completely. If possible, avoid all dairy and see if you are able to manage your disease without them.

Is the Paleo Diet okay for people with high blood pressure?

High blood pressure is nothing to take lightly. If left untreated, it can lead to heart attacks, strokes and kidney failure, just to mention a few of the serious health implications that accompany high blood pressure. The main benefit for individuals with high blood pressure while on the Paleo Diet is the low salt intake. However, the Paleo Diet should not be used to control high blood pressure alone. It is best to see a physician and continue any recommended medications in addition to adopting the Paleo Diet into your treatment plan.

Can a vegetarian use the Paleo Diet?

Because the Paleo Diet is omnivorous by nature, vegetarians can easily shun it. However, a vegetarian can still find plenty of healthy options within the Paleo Diet. First, eat eggs and lots of them. You are also allowed some seeds that can help fill your craving for grains. If you are a heavy pasta eater then try zucchini noodles and spaghetti squash instead of traditional pasta noodles. And don't forget about the unlimited amounts of fruits and vegetables that you can also consume to keep things colorful and creative.

Is the Paleo Diet okay for children?

The concern behind this question usually evolves around the high amounts of meat and the lack of dairy, which ultimately is a concern about the lack of calcium. For the same reasons as already discussed, the Paleo Diet is just as safe for children as it is for adults. Considering that most children's diets contain unhealthy amounts of soy, grains and sugars, the high amounts of fruits, vegetables and lean meats are highly beneficial for proper growth.

There are a few adjustments that need to be made if you are going to transition as a family into the Paleo lifestyle. Kids are (or at least should be) incredibly active. Because they are constantly burning energy they need plenty of carbohydrates to keep their bodies well fueled. If you are limiting the amount of carbohydrates you ingest, don't place your children on the same restrictions (unless they need to lose weight as well). Give them plenty of fruits and vegetables (even the starchy ones like bananas, sweet potatoes, squash) and plenty of grass-fed meats and poultry to keep them healthy and strong.

If you are concerned about the lack of calcium then you can try your hardest to feed them high-calcium vegetables, or you can make healthy bone broths and use them as the basis for soups, cauliflower rice and other dishes. You can even just feed the broth to your infant or make a yummy chicken soup.

Is the Paleo Diet hard to follow?

This is one of those questions that has to be answered yes…and no. The Paleo Diet is hard because for most of us it is completely changing the way that we eat. Just like any diet you have to give it a chance to work. That means more than a week on the diet - or two weeks - or three weeks. You are trying to reset your body and heal systems that have suffered abuse for decades due to unhealthy or "healthy" eating.

The Paleo Diet is also hard because it requires you to consciously think and plan ahead when it comes to food. Your days of heading through drive-thru on your lunch break are over. You will need to research and plan meals, regularly go to the market and grocery store and develop an arsenal of recipes to consistently follow the Paleo Diet.

Having said that, the Paleo Diet is easy because there's only one rule: eat healthy and clean foods. It takes the guesswork out of reading packaging labels and removes the frustration of counting calories, calculating points and figuring out if that pork chop is larger or smaller than your fist.

Chapter 6: Sticking to the Paleo Diet

Planning a roadmap for the Paleo Diet is just as important as the decision to begin. It's not something that you can dive into overnight; it takes preparation to make sure you have all of the necessary foods and tools that you need. Before you commit to going all Paleo, here are some tips for tackling the grocery store and restaurants as well as what it looks like to incorporate the Paleolithic lifestyle in a holistic way.

Grocery Shopping Tips

The next step to beginning the Paleo Diet is the process of food shopping. This is where it can get tricky as some of the ingredients are hard to find and the chances of finding affordable options all in one location is going to be hard. Here are some tips to help you get started with grocery shopping as well as information on where to find some of the products.

When you grocery shop for the Paleo Diet you will spend most of your time shopping the perimeter. If you've ever thought about the layout of your grocery store, most likely meat, produce and dairy are situated along the perimeter while the center-filled aisles contain all of the non-perishable goods, household and personal care products and frozen foods. Because your shopping list will consist mainly of produce and meat, you will most likely find yourself sticking to the outside circle of the grocery store.

Processed foods are readily available and cheap. High quality meats and produce are not. Because of this, the Paleo Diet is not considered inexpensive especially if trying to follow the diet as a family. This is why it's important to focus on sales and stock-up on items when they are cheap. If you can't afford grass-fed beef, free range poultry, cage-free eggs and organic produce, then all is not lost!

If you must purchase meat from the grocery store then be sure to trim the fat. When cows and lambs are eating grass in the meadow and allowed to graze and roam freely, their meat is full of nutrients and healthy fat. If, however, your meat has come from a slaughterhouse from cows that have been pumped with antibiotics and fed a grain diet, a lot of unhealthy stuff gets stored in their fat. So, if working with store bought meat trim away!

When it comes to produce it's best to follow the guidelines put forth by the Environmental Working Group (EWG). Each year the EWG publishes two lists. One is called the Dirty Dozen and the other is titled the Clean Fifteen. The reports are two lists that highlight the produce most prone to contain high amounts of pesticides and should be purchased organic (Dirty Dozen) and produce that is safe to consume without going organic as they contain very little amounts of pesticides (Clean Fifteen).

For the year 2013, the following fruits and vegetables made the list:

Dirty Dozen (ish)

1. Apples
2. Celery
3. Cherry Tomatoes
4. Cucumbers
5. Grapes
6. Hot Peppers
7. Nectarines
8. Peaches
9. Potatoes
10. Spinach
11. Strawberries
12. Sweet Bell Peppers
13. Kale/Collard Greens
14. Summer Squash

Clean Fifteen

1. Asparagus
2. Avocados
3. Cabbage
4. Cantaloupe
5. Sweet Corn
6. Eggplant
7. Grapefruit
8. Kiwi
9. Mangoes
10. Mushrooms
11. Onions
12. Papayas
13. Pineapple
14. Sweet Peas – frozen
15. Sweet Potatoes

It should be noted that this is just a guide. If you can afford some of the organic produce on the Dirty Dozen then that's wonderful! Even if you can't afford or find organic varieties of the items found on the Dirty Dozen the benefits of eating the fresh fruit or vegetable outweigh the risk of possible pesticides.

Well-Stocked Pantry

In addition to meat and produce, there are some pantry staples that you should always have on hand. Items like canned coconut milk, nuts, canned tomatoes, canned stocks, etc. are best purchased in bulk so that you always have them ready to go for those evenings when you get home late from work and need a meal fast. These are some of the items that can be harder to find.

If you are looking for coconut milk try to purchase full-fat milk. This way you get all of the healthy nutrients found in coconuts and you get your money's worth! Trader Joe's is a great place to purchase coconut milk. If shopping in your grocery store try looking in the Asian Foods aisle. You can also visit your local Asian Market to find coconut milk.

Trader Joe's also has affordable options for almond butter, boxed organic stocks and coconut oil. In addition, check your local health food store as well as online retailers to find the best and most affordable options. Remember that you are beginning a new diet and so it might take you a while to master the new way of shopping. Just schedule a little bit longer the first few weeks so that you can shop with plenty of time and not feel rushed in decision-making.

Eating Out On Paleo

When you begin to eat Paleo you will quickly notice how un-Paleo the restaurant world has become! It is loaded with salt, starches and low quality meats to offer us "high-quality" meals at low-prices. If you live in a metropolitan area it might be easier to find restaurants that feature grass-fed beef but for most of us eating out while trying to adhere to the Paleo Diet can seem impossible.

There are several options to overcome this problem. The first option is somewhat impractical. If there are not any Paleo options available then you just don't go out to eat. This can be challenging, especially if you are the primary cook in your household. Sometimes you just want a break from the chopping, mincing and sautéing! While a strict eat-in-only policy is good from time-to-time, it isn't really sustainable.

The second option to eating out while on Paleo is to choose restaurants that offer foods as close to Paleo as they come. You could order a Cobb salad, minus the dressing, croutons, etc., and instead drizzle oil and vinegar over the contents. If patronizing your local burger joint you could opt for a bun-less burger and or request lettuce leaves to make a wrap. This option does require some creative know-how but it can be done!

The final option is to view your restaurant meals as cheat days. This means that you follow the Paleo Diet as much as you can but allow yourself some leniency when dining out. Followers of the Paleo Diet often choose this option as eating the Paleo way can seem socially isolating. Because so much of our social interaction revolves around food it becomes cumbersome to be turning down special treats at friends' houses or forgoing heading out with co-workers because you can't eat anything on the menu! This option keeps your social life healthy and allows indulgence every once in a while.

The Paleolithic Lifestyle

Eating Paleo is just one of the many facets of the Paleolithic lifestyle. Another major area of focus for followers of the Paleo Diet is fitness. When looking back into the lives of our ancestors it's not just about food, adherents of the Paleo Diet are seeking transformation of the modern lifestyle that seems to foster unhealthy habits. One of those unhealthy habits is lack of exercise.

Although many followers of the diet consider themselves performance athletes, you do not have to bench press 300 lbs to be considered Paleo! The more exercise you can establish in your life, the better. Running, walking, yoga, Pilates, swimming, playing tag with your kids, all of these are beneficial and necessary for total health. In addition to low-strain exercise, it is also important to incorporate more strenuous exercise that is pushing the body to work harder and go farther. Activities like CrossFit and martial arts are excellent programs to learn.

The Paleo lifestyle also encompasses our periods of rest. One cannot underestimate the importance of sleep to live a healthy lifestyle. When we lay our heads on our pillows at night our minds might be resting but our bodies are still hard at work.

It is during sleep that our memories work to ingrain the messages and images that we've received throughout the day. Our ability to work the following day is largely due to the amount of sleep received the night before. This is especially true for children. Ironically, we are more prone to behavioral problems and hyperactivity when we do not have enough sleep. Overall, sleep is just good for the brain and body.

The final element of a Paleo lifestyle is community. Look for online forums and seek out members of your community that are also following the Paleo Diet. It can be hard to follow the diet in a vacuum but if others who have chosen this way of clean, healthy living surround you then you are already a step ahead in the game.

Some Tips to Get Started

Hopefully at this point you are excited and not too overwhelmed. Below are some useful tips to consider before going all-out Paleo. They will help you get started in the right direction and set you up for success from the very beginning:

1. Do a sweep of your entire house and eliminate all non-Paleo foods. You can throw them out, donate them to a local food bank or give them away to friends and neighbors. At the very least put all of the non-perishable items in a box and stick it in the top shelf of the pantry.

The idea is to start with a clean slate.

2. Plan ahead before you make the switch to a Paleo Diet. While getting up one morning and shouting, "I declare myself to be a Paleo eater!" sounds cool, you'll fail by lunch if you don't have a well-stocked pantry, fridge and freezer with all of those great foods.

3. Research to find some great Paleo recipes. At the end of this guide you'll find recipes and meal guides but don't let your exploration end there. There are countless websites to help keep variety in your Paleo diet.

4. Keep plenty of Paleo friendly beverages on hand like water, sparkling water and herbal teas. Because your body will likely go through a detoxification process it's important to stay well hydrated. If you start to feel hungry in-between meals try drinking before snacking.

5. Try to incorporate the entire family. If you have decided to eat Paleo but can't seem to convince your spouse, then keep trying! You need a support team as you change and become healthier and the best support team is your family.

Chapter 7: Meal plans and easy recipes

When you first begin eating the Paleo way it can be confusing to figure out what you can and cannot eat.   Following meal plans keeping an arsenal of recipes at hand are great ways to ease into the diet. Seeing as you are overhauling the way that you eat, trying to build a weekly food menu without any processed can be a challenge. While there's not a rulebook that states you must follow a sample meal plan or stick to Paleo specific recipes, they are available to make the transition easier.

Sample Meal Plan

The sample meal plan below contains a full week's worth of healthy Paleo Diet meals. It also includes an optional snack each day that you can eat or pass based on your hunger levels. Remember to stay well hydrated as you face your first week of Paleo, as much of your initial hunger will occur from the sugar detoxification process that is going on inside of your body.

Any recipes for the meal plan are located in the Paleo Diet Recipes section at the end of the chapter. To create a full meal plan, there are no repeats or days marked "leftovers". It is completely realistic that you will have lunches that consist of leftovers from dinner but a weekly meal plan without any repeats or leftovers gives you a better idea of the awesome variety that you can find while eating Paleo.

Day	Breakfast	Lunch	Dinner	Snack
Monday	Paleo Pancakes	Prosciutto Wrapped Egg Muffins	Burgers with Sweet Potato Buns	Berries with Coconut Shavings
Tuesday	Sausage Omelet	Wilted Kale Salad	Almond Chicken With Mushroom Sauce	Lettuce Wrapped Vegetable Sticks
Wednesday	Scrambled Eggs and Sweet Potato Hash	Paleo Cobb Salad	Curry with Fish and Vegetables	Apples with Almond Butter
Thursday	Ground Beef, Apples & Cinnamon	Chicken Lettuce Wraps	Paleo Chili	Kale Chips with Balsamic Vinegar and Oil
Friday	Coconut Oatmeal Paleo Style	Paleo Spaghetti	Zucchini and Ground Beef Stir-Fry	Paleo Hummus
Saturday	Scrambled Eggs with Avocado and Bacon	Grilled Meat Kebabs	Stuffed Peppers	Paleo Candy Bars
Sunday	Smoked Salmon and	Grilled Chicken Breasts with	Pork With Fennel and	Ants On A Log

Breakfast Recipes

1. Paleo Pancakes

Yields: 1 serving

Ingredients:

1 tbsp. Almond Butter
2 Ripe Bananas
1 Egg

Directions:

1. Blend all ingredients until smooth.
2. Heat coconut oil in griddle.
3. Pour ½ butter onto griddle and brown each side. Repeat.
4. Serve with fresh fruit, if desired.

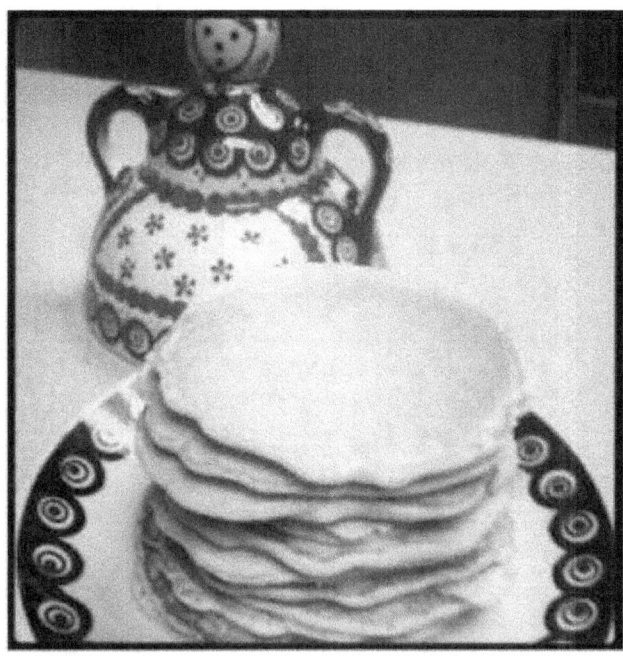

Cooking Cinderella/CookingCinderella/Flickr
http://www.flickr.com/photos/81884868@N07/8557696060/

2. Sausage Omelet

Yields: 1 serving

Ingredients:

2 eggs
½ lb. cooked nitrate free pork sausage
Fresh chopped parsley (optional)

Directions:

1. Heat approximately 1 tsp of coconut oil in medium skillet.
2. Beat the eggs and add to skillet.
3. Once eggs start to set, sprinkle sausage on one half of the eggs and fold over the other half.
4. Flip until the other side is fully cooked.
5. Sprinkle with parsley, if desired.

3. Scrambled Eggs and Sweet Potato Hash

Yields: 2 servings

Ingredients:

4-6 eggs
1 large sweet potato, peeled and shredded
Cayenne pepper to taste
Chopped green onions

Directions:

1. Heat 4 tbsp. coconut oil in large skillet.
2. Lay the shredded sweet potato in the skillet in an even layer.
3. Let cook for 15 minutes until bottom is crispy, then flip.
4. Continue to cook until the other side is brown and crisp.
5. Once cooked, remove from pan and heat 1 tsp coconut oil.
6. Add eggs to the pan and cook until the yolks have reached desired consistency (or scramble the eggs).

7. Divide potato hash onto two plates and top with eggs. Sprinkle with cayenne pepper and green onions to taste.

4. Ground Beef, Apples & Cinnamon

Yields: 2-3 servings

Ingredients:

1 lb. ground beef
2 medium apples, diced
1 tsp. cinnamon
Salt and pepper

Directions:

1. In a medium skillet cook the ground beef until just a little pink is visible.
2. Add the apples and cinnamon to the pan and cook until apples are crisp-tender. Season with salt and pepper if desired.
3. Divide the meat mixture between 2-3 plates and enjoy!

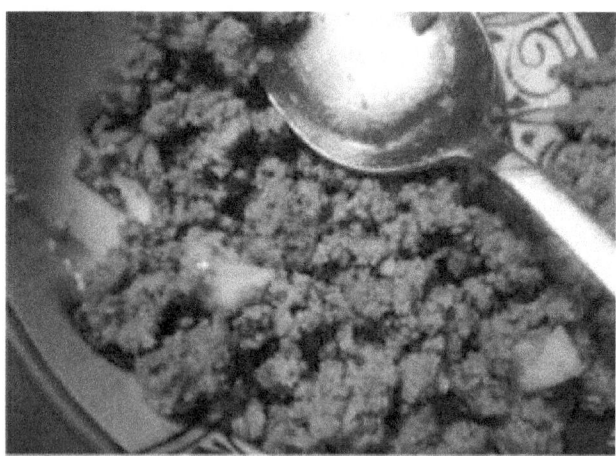

anasararojas/Flickr
http://www.flickr.com/photos/anasararojas/6809424077/

5. Coconut Oatmeal Paleo Style

Yields: 1 serving

Ingredients:

2/3 cup coconut milk (unsweetened)
¼ cup unsweetened shredded coconut
1 tsp vanilla
2 tbsp. almond meal or almond flour
1 tbsp. flaxseed meal (optional)
Honey (optional)
Fresh fruit (optional)

Directions:
1. Heat the coconut milk in a small saucepan.
2. Add remaining ingredients and cook until slightly thick.
3. Top with honey and fruit, if desired, and enjoy!

6. **Scrambled Eggs with Avocado and Bacon**

    Yields: 2 servings

    Ingredients:

    4-6 eggs, beaten
    2 ripe avocadoes, peeled, seeded and diced
    2-4 slices of nitrate free bacon cut into small strips

    Directions:

    1. Heat medium skillet and add bacon, turning until fully cooked.
    2. Remove the bacon and remove out all but 1tsp of the bacon grease left in the pan (be sure and save the fat for future meals).
    3. Pour egg mixture into pan and stir until fully cooked, scraping any pieces off of the bottom of the pan.
    4. Divide egg mixture between two plates and sprinkle with avocado and bacon.

7. **Smoked Salmon and Fried Eggs**

    Yields: 2 servings

Ingredients:

10 oz. smoked salmon
4-6 eggs, beaten

Directions:

1. Heat 1 tbsp. coconut oil in medium skillet.
2. Add eggs and stir until just set.
3. Add smoked salmon to the skillet and stir until heated through.
4. Divide between two plates and serve.

Lunch Recipes

1. **Prosciutto Wrapped Egg Muffins**

    Yields: 6 muffins

    Ingredients:

    ½ onion, diced
    2 cloves garlic, minced
    Handful of mushrooms, chopped
    Handful of fresh spinach, chopped
    8 large eggs
    ¼ cup coconut milk
    2 tbsp. coconut flour
    5 ounces Prosciutto

    Directions:

    1. Preheat the oven to 375°.

    2. Heat coconut oil in skillet and add garlic and mushrooms until vegetables are crisp tender. Add spinach and season with salt and pepper. Cook for 3-5 minutes longer.

    3. In a large bowl, beat eggs, coconut milk, coconut flour, salt and pepper until ingredients are well blended. Add vegetable mixture to the bowl and stir.

4. Brush each muffin cup with melted coconut oil and then completely line the sides and bottom with prosciutto.
5. Spoon the egg batter evenly throughout the six muffin cups.
6. Cook in the oven for 20-25 minutes until the mixture is nice and fluffy.
7. Remove from muffin pan and cool.

2. Wilted Kale Salad

Yields: 2-3 servings

Ingredients:

1 bunch kale, chopped
Handful of raspberries
1 lb. nitrate free bacon, chopped
Handful of pine nuts or chopped almonds

Directions:

1. Place kale, raspberries and chopped nuts into a large bowl. Set aside.
2. Heat a medium skillet and add bacon, stirring until bacon is fully cooked.
3. Pour bacon and grease into bowl and toss until kale is completely covered.
4. Cover bowl for 5 minutes, allowing the kale to wilt.
5. Sprinkle with salt and pepper and serve.

3. Paleo Cobb Salad

Yields: 2-3 servings

Ingredients:

2-3 romaine lettuce leave heads, chopped
4-6 pieces of nitrate free bacon, chopped
3 eggs
1 medium tomato, chopped
1 bunch green onions, chopped
2 tbsp. sliced almonds

Balsamic Vinegar
Olive Oil
Salt & Pepper

Directions:

1. Place eggs in a medium saucepan and cover with water.
2. Place saucepan on the stove and bring to a boil.
3. Once boiling, cover the saucepan and remove from heat. Let eggs sit in hot water for 12 minutes.
4. While eggs are cooking, heat a medium skillet and add bacon, stirring frequently until bacon is fully cooked.
5. Place chopped lettuce, tomato, green onions and sliced almonds into a large bowl. Stir all ingredients together.
6. Remove bacon from pan and add to lettuce mix. Divide lettuce mixture between 2-3 plates.
7. Once eggs are finished, peel and slice, adding one egg to each salad.
8. Drizzle salads with balsamic vinegar, olive, salt and pepper to taste.

4. Chicken Lettuce Wraps

Yields: 3-4 servings

Ingredients:

1 lb. ground chicken (or pork, or beef)
5 oz. mushrooms, finely diced
1/3 cup scallions, chopped
3 cloves garlic, minced
1 tbsp. sesame oil
¼ cup slivered or sliced almonds
3 tbsp. coconut oil
3 tbsp. honey
2 tbsp. water
½ cup coconut aminos
3 tbsp. vinegar
Hot Sauce
Salt and Pepper

Romaine or Bibb lettuce leaves
Shredded carrots and cabbage

Directions:

1. Heat the coconut oil in a large pan. Add chicken to the pan and cook through, seasoning with salt and pepper to taste.
2. Add mushrooms, scallions, garlic, almonds and sesame oil to pan.
3. Mix together honey, water, coconut aminos and vinegar. Add mixture to pan and cook until heated through.
4. Remove from pan and spoon into lettuce leaves. Top with carrots and cabbage to serve.
5. Have hot sauce available to sprinkle on top.

5. Paleo Spaghetti

Yields: 3-4 servings

Ingredients:

1 medium size spaghetti squash
1.5-2 lbs. ground beef
1 onion, diced
3 cloves garlic, minced
2 (8 oz.) cans tomato sauce
1 (28 oz.) can diced tomatoes, drained
1 (6 oz.) can Tomato Paste
Fresh basil
Fresh Oregano
Salt and Pepper

Directions:

1. Preheat oven to 375°.
2. Cut the spaghetti squash in half lengthwise.
3. Scrape out the seeds and pulp.
4. Lay the squash halves in a 13x9 baking dish, rind side facing up.

5. Bake for 30-40 minutes or until you can easily pierce the rind with a knife.
6. When spaghetti squash is thoroughly cooked, scrape the pulp out with a fork, creating strands that resemble spaghetti noodles.
7. While the squash is cooking, place the ground beef, garlic and onion in a large skillet. Cooked until lightly browned.
8. Add tomato sauce, diced tomatoes and tomato paste. Let simmer for 15 minutes.
9. Add fresh basil, oregano and salt and pepper to taste.
10. Serve over spaghetti sauce.

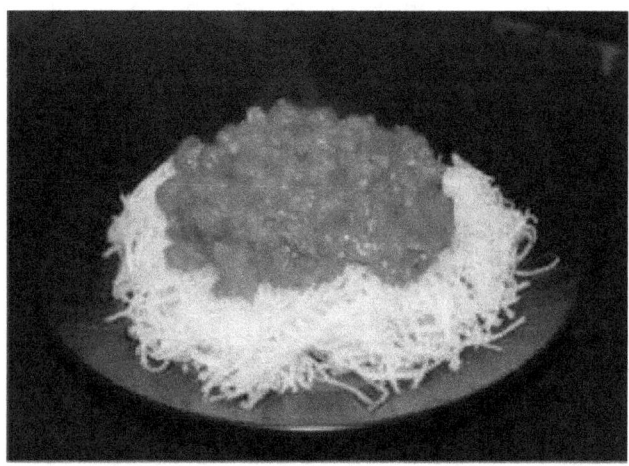

Scott Veg/Thriving Vegetarian/Flickr
http://www.flickr.com/photos/thrivingveg/8542529328/

6. Grilled Meat Kebabs

Yields: 3-4 servings

Ingredients:

1 lb. meat cubed (steak, chicken, or pork)
½ cup olive oil
4 cloves garlic, minced
1 teaspoon oregano
1 teaspoon thyme
1 onion sliced in large chunks

8 ounce carton of whole mushrooms
3 bell peppers sliced in large chunks
2 medium tomatoes sliced into large chunks
Fresh pineapple (optional) cut into large chunks

Directions:

1. Combine the olive oil, garlic oregano and thyme into a large freezer bag. Add the meat and shake to thoroughly coat.
2. Let meat marinate overnight in refrigerator (ideal) or at least hour if you are rushed.
3. Using metal or bamboo skewers, alternate meat and vegetables onto the skewers. Or, you can create meat only kebabs and vegetable only kebabs.
4. If desired, create pineapple skewers to serve alongside the meat and vegetables.
5. Grill over medium high heat until meat is cooked and vegetables are crisp tender. Pineapple skewers only need to be grilled a few minutes on each side.

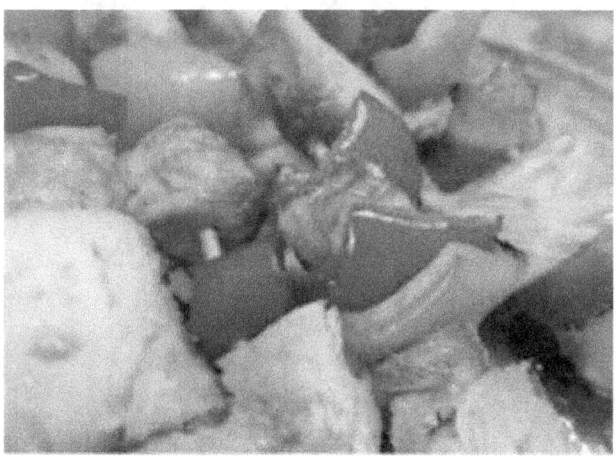

Micah Sittig/Micah Sittig/Flicker
http://www.flickr.com/photos/msittig/4802237416/

7.   Grilled Chicken Breasts

Yields: 4 servings

Ingredients:

4 boneless, skinless chicken breasts
¼ cup olive oil
¼ cup balsamic vinegar
2-3 garlic cloves, minced
1 tbsp. fresh basil
Salt and Pepper

Directions:

1. Place olive oil, balsamic vinegar, garlic and basil into a freezer bag. Add salt and pepper if desired.
2. Add chicken and shake to coat.
3. Refrigerate overnight or at least 2 hours if pressed for time.
4. Grill until chicken is thoroughly cooked.

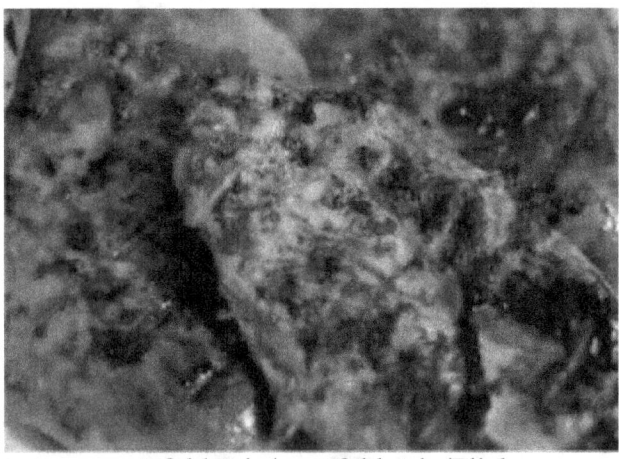

scott feldstein/scottfeldstein/Flickr
http://www.flickr.com/photos/scottfeldstein/405368402/

Dinner Recipes

1. **Pork with fennel and bacon**

    Yields: 4 servings

Ingredients:

4 pork chops
1.5 cups full fat cream
1 fennel bulb, thinly sliced
4 slices of nitrate free bacon, thinly sliced
1 small onion, thinly sliced
2 garlic cloves, minced
Salt and Pepper

Directions:

1. Preheat oven to 350°.
2. Place pork chops in shallow cooking dish, sprinkle with salt and pepper and cook for 30-45 minutes.
3. While pork is cooking, heat bacon in a medium saucepan, stirring frequently, until bacon is about half-cooked.
4. Add fennel, onion and garlic, stirring until vegetables are tender.
5. Pour cream into pan and heat through.
6. Serve cream sauce over pork chops.

2. Stuffed Peppers

Yields: 3-4 servings

Ingredients:

4 large bell peppers, any color
1 lb. ground meat or poultry
2 cups cauliflower, riced
8 oz. can tomato sauce
½ cup onions, chopped into fine pieces
2 tbsp. coconut oil
2 tbsp. garlic, minced
½ tsp red pepper flakes
¼ tsp cayenne pepper (if desired)
Salt and pepper to taste

Directions:

1. Preheat oven to 350°.

2. In a large stew pot, bring 6 cups water to boil.
3. Remove seeds and membranes from pepper. Place peppers in the pot and boil for one minute to blanch.
4. Remove peppers and set aside to cool.
5. In a medium saucepan, heat coconut oil. Add onions, garlic and cauliflower rice, stirring until onions are translucent.
6. In a separate bowl, combine meat, red pepper flakes, cayenne pepper, tomato sauce, salt and pepper.
7. Add onion mixture to meat mixture and stir until combined.
8. Divide the mixture equally among the peppers and place in shallow oven dish.
9. Cook for 35-45 minutes or until meat is cooked through.

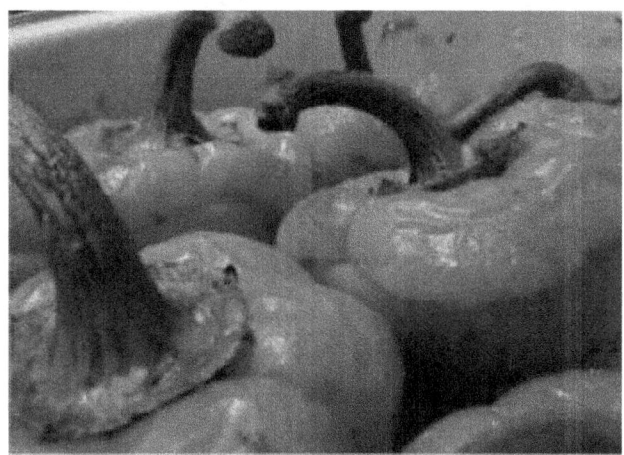

ella/ella novak/Flickr
http://www.flickr.com/photos/cookylida/5591197517/

3. Zucchini, Mushrooms and Ground Beef Stir-Fry

Yields: 3-4 servings

Ingredients:

1 medium zucchini, diced
8 oz carton of mushrooms, sliced
1 lb. ground beef

1 tbsp. coconut oil
Salt and pepper

Directions:

1. Heat coconut oil in a medium skillet.
2. Add ground beef and cook until meat is barely browned.
3. Add zucchini and mushrooms, cooking until vegetables are crisp tender.
4. Season to taste.

4. **Paleo chili**

Yields: 8-10 servings

Ingredients:

2 lbs. ground beef
1 tbsp. coconut oil
1.5 cups chopped onion
1 green bell pepper, chopped
4 cloves garlic, minced
28 oz. can diced tomatoes, undrained
28 oz. can crushed tomatoes
8 oz. cans tomato sauce
1 Tbs. chili powder
Dried basil
2 bay leaves
Dried oregano
Crushed red pepper flakes
Salt and pepper

Directions:

1. In a large stewpot, heat coconut oil. Add onion, garlic and bell pepper to pot.
2. Stir for a few minutes and then add ground beef.
3. Once mixture is browned, add diced tomatoes, crushed tomatoes, tomato sauce, and all seasonings to taste.

4. Cover and let simmer for 20-30 minutes, tasting occasionally and adding seasoning as needed.
5. Garnish with avocado, cilantro, jalapenos, etc.

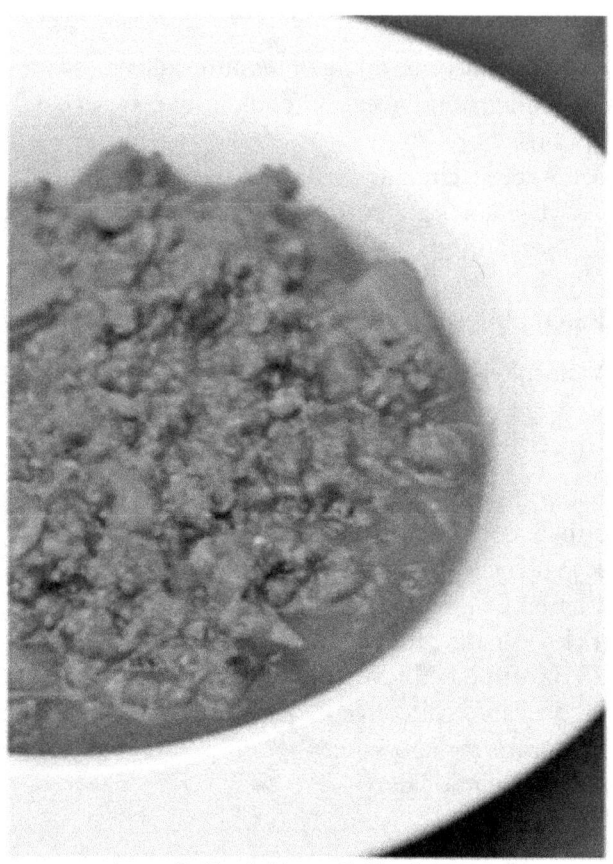

Amy Selleck/AmySelleck/Flickr
http://www.flickr.com/photos/amyselleck/5012092911/

5. Curry with fish and vegetables

Yields: 2-3 servings

Ingredients:

4-5 white fish fillets
4 medium tomatoes, chopped
2 bell peppers (any color), chopped
1 8 oz package mushrooms, chopped
2 zucchinis, chopped

13.5 oz can coconut milk
2 tbsp. dried ginger
3-4 cloves garlic, finely chopped
6 tbsp. fish sauce
3 tsp cumin
¾ tsp turmeric
4 teaspoons honey (optional)
Salt and pepper (optional)
Lemon juice (optional)

Directions:

1. In a medium saucepan, bring 3 cups of water to a boil. Add fish and cook until fish flakes easily with a fork.
2. Flake fish into small pieces within the water.
3. Add vegetables and boil until crisp tender.
4. Add coconut milk, ginger, garlic, fish sauce, cumin, turmeric, honey, salt and pepper.
5. Cook until mixture is heated through. Taste and season accordingly.

6. Almond chicken with mushroom sauce

Yields: 4 servings

Ingredients:

4 chicken breasts, tenderized if too thick
½ cup almond meal
½ tsp garlic powder
½ tsp tarragon
¼ tsp paprika
Salt and pepper
¼ cup coconut oil
¼ cup dry sherry (optional)
¾ cup coconut milk
8 oz carton of mushrooms, sliced

Directions:

1. In a shallow plate, combine almond meal, garlic powder, tarragon, paprika, salt and pepper.

2. Coat chicken breasts in flour mixture, shaking off any excess.
3. Heat coconut oil in a large skillet and add chicken breasts to pan.
4. Cook approximately 5 minutes each side (or longer if meat is still pink).
5. Remove chicken from pan and set aside.
6. Slowly pour dry sherry into pan, scraping up any brown bits. Add mushrooms and cook until soft.
7. Add coconut milk and cook until heated through. Serve sauce over chicken breasts.

7. Burgers with sweet potato buns

Yields: 4 servings

Ingredients:

1 lb. ground beef
2 large sweet potatoes, peeled and cut into thick slices
2 ½ tbsp. paprika
2 tbsp. garlic powder
2 tsp ground mustard
1 tsp cayenne pepper
Olive Oil Cumin
Salt and Pepper

Directions:

1. Preheat oven to 350□.
2. Place ground beef into a medium bowl and sprinkle with paprika, garlic powder, ground mustard, cayenne pepper, salt and pepper to taste.
3. Using your fingers, mix the spices throughout the ground beef and form into four patties. Set aside.
4. Place sweet potato slices into a large bowl and drizzle with olive oil, salt, pepper and cumin to taste.
5. Lay potato slices on a shallow baking dish. Cook for 10-15 minutes per side, until a fork can easily pierce potatoes.

6. While potatoes are cooking, heat a medium skillet. Place patties onto skillet and heat, turning occasionally until desired temperature is reached.
7. Serve patties sandwiched in-between sweet potato slices.

Snack Recipes

1. Berries with Coconut Shavings

Yields: 1 serving

Ingredients:

½ cup mixed berries
2 tbsp. unsweetened coconut flakes

Directions:

Sprinkle mixed berries with unsweetened coconut flakes and enjoy!

2. Lettuce wrapped vegetable sticks

Yields: 1 serving

Ingredients:

½ carrots cut into small matchstick slices
½ zucchini cut into small matchstick slices
1 celery stalk cut into small matchstick slices
Romaine or Bibb lettuce
Balsamic Vinegar
Olive Oil

Directions:

Place desired portion of vegetables into lettuce and wrap lettuce around the vegetables. Dip in oil and vinegar.

3. Paleo candy bars (for an occasional treat)

Yields: 6-10 servings

Ingredients:

4 tbsp. coconut oil
¼ cup cocoa
½ cup almond meal
¾ cups dried, shredded unsweetened coconut
2-3 tbsp. honey (optional)

Directions:

1. In a medium sauce melt coconut oil and honey.
2. Remove from heat and add cocoa, almond meal and unsweetened coconut.
3. Place by spoonfuls onto a baking sheet lined with parchment paper and refrigerate or freeze until hardened.

4. Kale Chips

Yields: 4 servings

Ingredients:

1 bunch kale
2 tbsp. olive oil
Salt and pepper

Directions:

1. Preheat oven to 275°.
2. Remove the ribs from each kale stem and break kale into 1.5 inch pieces.
3. Place the kale pieces onto a baking sheet and sprinkle with oil, salt and pepper.
4. Bake about 20 minutes, turning halfway.

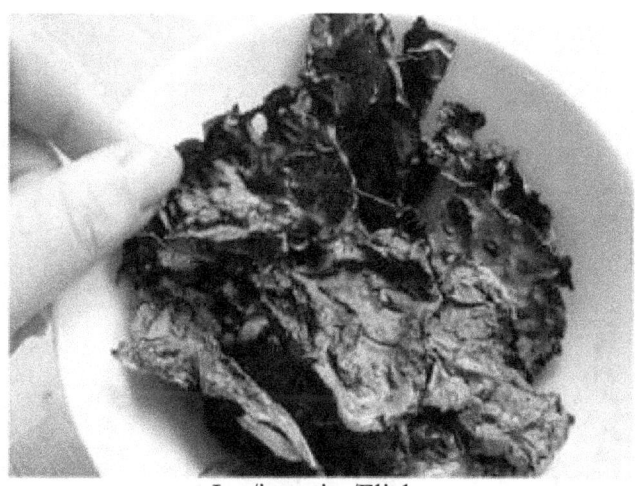

Joy/joyosity/Flickr
http://www.flickr.com/photos/joyosity/3322910677/

5. **Apples with almond butter**

Yields: 1 serving

Ingredients:

1 apple cut into slices

¼ cup almond butter

Directions:

Dip apples into almond butter and enjoy!

6. **Paleo Hummus**

Yields: 3-4 servings

Ingredients:
1 ¾ cup zucchini, peeled and cut into small pieces
½ cup raw, unsalted macadamia nuts
2 tbsp. olive oil
2 tbsp. tahini
2 garlic cloves
Sea Salt
1 tsp cumin
Dash of cayenne pepper

Directions:

Place all ingredients into a food processor or blender and blend until well combined. Sprinkle with paprika to garnish and enjoy!

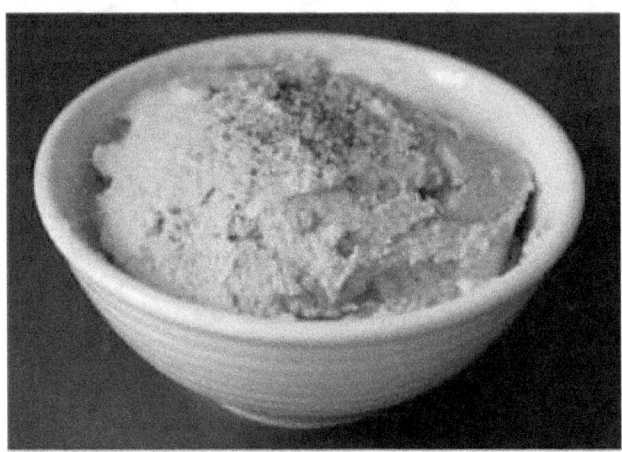

Whitney/whitneyinchicago/Flickr
http://www.flickr.com/photos/whitneyinchicago/

7. Ants On A Log Paleo style

Yields: 1 serving

Ingredients:

Celery stalks, rinsed and cut into 6-inch slices
Almond butter
Raisins

Directions:
Spoon almond butter into celery stalks, top with raisins and enjoy!